SLEEP IS NOW A FOREIGN COUNTRY

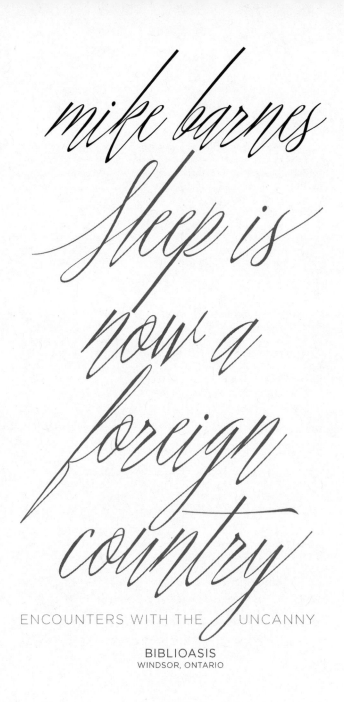

mike barnes

sleep is now a foreign country

ENCOUNTERS WITH THE UNCANNY

BIBLIOASIS
WINDSOR, ONTARIO

FIRST EDITION

10 9 8 7 6 5 4 3 2 1

Library and Archives Canada Cataloguing in Publication

Title: Sleep is now a foreign country : encounters with the uncanny / Mike Barnes.
Names: Barnes, Mike, 1955– author.
Identifiers: Canadiana (print) 2022047432X | Canadiana (ebook) 20220474370 | ISBN 9781771965125 (softcover) | ISBN 9781771965132 (EPUB)
Subjects: LCSH: Barnes, Mike, 1955– | CSH: Authors, Canadian (English)—20th century—Biography. | LCGFT: Autobiographies.
Classification: LCC PS8553.A7633 Z46 2023 | DDC C818/.5403—dc23

Edited by Daniel Wells
Copyedited by John Sweet
Cover and text designed by Ingrid Paulson

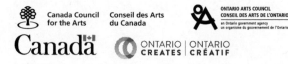

Published with the generous assistance of the Canada Council for the Arts, which last year invested $153 million to bring the arts to Canadians throughout the country, and the financial support of the Government of Canada. Biblioasis also acknowledges the support of the Ontario Arts Council (OAC), an agency of the Government of Ontario, which last year funded 1,709 individual artists and 1,078 organizations in 204 communities across Ontario, for a total of $52.1 million, and the contribution of the Government of Ontario through the Ontario Book Publishing Tax Credit and Ontario Creates.

PRINTED AND BOUND IN CANADA

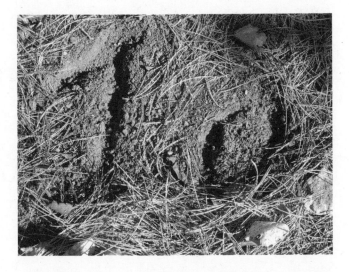

Food in dreams appears to be the same as food when awake,
but the sleepers are asleep, and receive no nourishment.
—Augustine, *Confessions*

On a spring afternoon in 2007, I was lying on the couch
in my living room reading *Simon Schama's Power of Art*.
This chapter was an essay on Picasso's *Guernica*. As I read
Schama's account of the German planes appearing in the
sky over the Spanish town on April 26, 1937, something
caused me to look up from the book. The objects in the

room, clearly outlined in the spring light, seemed altered somehow, stark yet dubious along their edges. Not quite familiar, either as themselves or as an arrangement of objects. I had a sense of items poised in a museum, absorbing my attention while contriving to escape it utterly. Clear and hunkered as they were, I couldn't quite see them. I realized then the date was April 26. The same day as the Guernica attack, exactly seventy years later.

The bombers had appeared in the sky at 4 p.m. I looked at the homemade wooden clock on the end table. Hand-sawed and painted yellow-green, it has the shape of a tall, slim house with no window and, at its base, a little red door askew on its hinges. The hour hand had dropped below the eave on the right, two-thirds of its way toward the crooked little door. The big hand pointed straight up into the peak of the tall roof. It was 4 p.m.

For a long instant, like the sustained vibrations of a musical chord, past and present collapsed together like the two ends of an accordioned paper figure. Or more than two: the moment thronged with splintery harmonics. Stretched out, the two sequences—the destruction of a town, which became the subject of a famous painting, which became the subject of an essay; and (reversing things) my reading of the essay about the painting about the destroyed town—were separated by the innumerable twists and folds of seven decades. Then somehow, with a speed that gave me vertigo, they shut up tight together, without a wafer of space between them.

They overlaid each other like clear transparencies. That was part of the vertigo. As if the intervening seventy years had suddenly gone sheer and negligible. Like wandering (I was looking at the house-clock again) in a building made of glass. A glass construction polished to such speckless transparency that things which ordinary walls and floors and ceilings would keep apart could suddenly loom, merge and blend.

But there was movement in that image. There had to be. In part to account for the lurching, jittery sense I felt lying there. A sense of caged turbulence—wild whirling bounded by absolute stillness—like the frenzy of snowflakes inside a glass-globed paperweight.

A dance, I thought. In a dance you whirl through space without ever leaving the dance. At a given moment someone may be across the ballroom, or right next to you, or in your arms—these positions and others can repeat and alternate. All of these thoughts and comparisons, none of them quite right, none of them exactly wrong, could go on without any disruption to the dance itself. Perhaps they were even part of it. A step, a style of stepping, however ungainly, that I could claim and recognize as my own.

For if the pure exhilaration of this kind of dancing has always come with close echoes of apprehensiveness, it is not just because of its weightlessness and the transparency of its figures, those unmoored, glassy possibilities that bring havoc just as easily as redemption to the world of solid sense and obscurity. It is because, once finding myself aswirl again, I have never had the slightest clue when or where or how the dance will end.

. . .

After that, there was nothing for a few days. Then the first transmissions, widely spaced. The number 70. Lines and circles scratched in dirt. My grandfather's face. These could be core signals, or peripheral or preliminary, perhaps to test or clear the line. There was no way to tell at this point. I knew by now to do nothing but wait.

. . .

In July 1963, John "Jack" Green, my grandfather on my mom's side, died suddenly of a heart attack, aged seventy. I was seven, almost eight, at the time. Ever since then, his death, as Mom described it to me, has been the model in my mind of a "good death." The sort of swift and summing exit not granted to many. He was a gentle, churchgoing man, worn but not broken by working a Saskatchewan wheat farm for fifty years, including the worst years of the Depression. His father had been one of the first eastern settlers to build on the land outside Boharm. On the last day of his life, my grandfather came in from the field to have lunch with his wife. He was still vigorous, still active in the pattern of his days. "I feel tired, Maudie," he said as he settled into his chair. "I'm just going to close my eyes for a bit." When my grandmother came back from the kitchen, he was gone. Sitting with his eyes still closed, his hands still folded; no signs of pain or panic. As if, having reached his Biblical allotment of threescore and ten, he was permitted to depart peacefully, like a ploughman who has faithfully cut the long furrows back and forth in a vast field and can now, having reached the far corner, leave the implement and slip into some nearby shade for his rest.[1]

But similes, like everything else, depend for their meanings on the frame that bounds them, on how far they're allowed to go. Meaning is a bonsai operation. If the ploughman image is permitted to extend even slightly, there is, for the one back in the farmhouse, the matter of the abandoned plough, which must be dealt with, and the mystery of the vanished labourer. My grandmother, Maude,

---

1 Once, he sent me an arrowhead he'd found in a furrow. Busy as he was, he took the time to nestle the artifact in cotton batting in a little box and to write a description of how an Indian hunting buffalo might have lost it many decades, even centuries, before. It was a perfect arrowhead: notched at the base, whitish as if frosted on one side, semi-translucent on the other. For years it was my most prized possession: kept in its box by my bed, where I could inspect it daily. One day it disappeared. Stolen, obviously. My family speculated about the small number of suspects who had access to my room. But, though I mourned the loss, I had no interest in identifying the thief. Already I knew that there were holes in the fabric of life through which things slipped unaccountably—reality a sieve whose mesh could gape abruptly before compacting again. I barely thought of the theft in human terms. When I did conjecture about who might have robbed me, I felt, more than anger, a kind of queasy coziness. Certain thefts constitute an increase in intimacy, an unasked-for gloss by others on our lives. Ordinary rip-offs and pilferings, even online "identity theft," are not the activities of the Close Thief, as I came to call the arrowhead stealer. This Thief does not acquire, but *proceeds from*, intimate knowledge of who you are, what you value most. I have lost three possessions to the Thief: the arrowhead from my grandfather, a beaver skull I found on a beach, and a German edition of the poems of Charles Bukowski, which, apart from a tourist brochure of the Blautopf (see below), was my only tangible connection to the time I spent in Germany before going insane. In each case—instances spanning about fifteen years—the Close Thief went for the artifacts I clung to most dependently, vestiges of a vanished natural and personal history.

whose maiden name of Bastedo reveals her Spanish ancestry, had to wait eighteen years to follow Jack. Sighing, more frequently as the years passed, she would say, "I'm tired. I want to see Jack again." Or, "I'm ready to see Jack." Her hint of exasperation at the length of the vigil she was being taxed with in no way contradicted her legendary Christian faith, cheer and kindness to others. It made these qualities shine even brighter, as the foil of stoical resignation in which these gems sparkled. She continued shopping and cooking for the sick; volunteering at the church; telephoning and writing her seven children; sending each of her two dozen grandchildren a card with a note of love and a green dollar bill on our birthdays—*like Maudie* meant *good* in the family lexicon. Her death was as sudden and in-stride as Jack's. Literally in-stride in her case, as her heart gave out while she was walking home from church, struck down, as Jack had been, while active, while attending to what she loved and believed in. She had called all her children on the telephone the night before. The first time since Jack's death, they realized at the funeral, that she had phoned all seven of them on the same night. Several of them had heard her say, "I'm tired, I miss Jack," as close to a declaration of impatience as she came. The yoking of "tired" with the certainty of a glad reunion makes of death a falling asleep, but also a waking into the better world that her faith assured her would be waiting. Leaving a muddled waking dream, which, even to someone of Maude's devotion, the cheerfully executed but repetitive rounds of her long widowhood must have seemed sometimes, to awake in a perfected dream, lucid and permanent.

I remember, on that spring night in 1981, crossing the kitchen to where Mom stood with her back turned after replacing the phone in its cradle. She faced the corner, her shoulders furled with the start of grief. Then, my only thought was to comfort her as best I could. Now, though, looking back, I think beyond that moment to the story she would soon begin murmuring, of the closure of her mother's long vigil, like the dangling end of a long necklace or locket chain that had finally found its clasp. And I think, too, of my own situations in 1963 and 1981, and find differences and parallels, which sometimes switch about and become each other. At almost-eight, in 1963, I was about to enter grade three in a new home in a new city. Eighteen years later, I was living in a small room downtown (I had walked up the escarpment stairs to have dinner that evening), washing pots in a hospital kitchen by day, writing poems by night. I wrote and read and walked much of the night, sometimes skipping sleep to have a last coffee near the kitchen before my shift started at 6 a.m. I wrote on average several poems a night and mailed them to magazines around the world, which in turn mailed almost all of them back. More than happy, I felt awake. Finally awake—as if my whole life before psychosis had been a fever dream I tossed in, a swampy swirl of lulls and jolts that had had to accelerate to a climax before the fever could break and my eyes open.

Grandma Green was the last of my grandparents to die; her death closed the clasp of that generation. Grandpa and Grandma Barnes, residents of an Ottawa nursing home, had died, a few months apart, in 1977–78. I was in hospital at the time—often catatonic, I have been told and have no reason to doubt—and remember nothing of their passing. When I was discharged finally, in 1979, those two elderly people I had visited as a child were simply not there anymore. The photographs of their gravestones declared an absence without making it real. It was as if, while I was "away," my grandparents had been abducted by aliens and whisked to another planet. That was how it might have happened in the sci-fi books I had devoured in my early teens. Interplanetary agents might have been left behind to plant evidence explaining the disappearances. Such stories no longer held allure for me. For some years now I had been living a life replete with inexplicable transports and lacunae. The aliens were here, their work was everywhere. Except that I no longer believed in aliens. Or perhaps it is truer to say they no longer interested me. Their myriad crazy doings had exhausted me into indifference. I was drawn now to "realistic" authors, though their realism was for me a risky realm. Authors who wrote of characters whose lives evolved by discoverable cause and effect, linked chains of relationships and events, remembered as a chronological continuity — these authors, who were in the majority as I discovered, wrote tales no less fantastic than those of Heinlein or Philip K. Dick, but for far higher stakes. Those stakes were nothing less than the establishment and maintenance of an order of ordinarily fathomable life. An audacious goal. A hopeful and necessary one, it seemed to me, crucial and even heroic. At other times I found it deluded, craven, even obscene. My reactions to realistic fiction were extreme because its stakes, for me, were extreme. They were, in fact, ultimate. I needed to believe, despite overwhelming evidence to the contrary, that my own life followed discernible patterns, that events happened for reasons and that similarly solid people with their own evident trajectories—rather than phantoms whose visitations were random and unknowable—intersected with it. That personality was more than a series of fleetingly persuasive poses or mirages. My favourite authors gave the devil his due. Their fictions allowed for unexplained personal obsessions and drives, random and even magical occurrences, but they incorporated these irruptions into a skein of narrative causality. Knut Hamsun, Brian Moore, J.G. Ballard, Isaac Singer. Emotions like meteor showers; fluctuating spells of death and apparitions of the Virgin Mary; the world's cities sunk in deep lagoons, a car crash love cult; dybbuks and succubi and eunuchs mad by the full moon—but between these marvels, admitting but also denying them implicitly, the linked words and phrases of plausible action, reaction, sentence after sentence, page after page. The world of sense; of linked, constituent parts. A tractable creation. A submitted one.[2]

The pine tree. Chedoke Public School, when I started there in the fall of 1963, first placed me in a grade two classroom instead of grade three. We had moved to Hamilton in the summer and perhaps my records from the old school were mixed up or delayed. In any case, what cracked Mom up when she told the story was the interval of several days during which I kept silent about being in the wrong grade. When I did speak up, I burst into tears, all my throttled misery spilling out at once. But she found curious, and perhaps a little appalling (her laughter had a nervous edge), the time when I kept *stumm* about my demotion. Taking my seat in the out-of-date classroom, conscientiously completing last year's work. She found that remarkable. I find it typical, and an augury of sorts. I would have kept quiet partly from timidity, but also from a conviction, which dates back as far as I can remember, that all powers are

---

2 In those early days out on the street again, my writing diet was more omnivorous than my reading one. Mixed in with poems on rivers and rain, scrambled eggs and street fights over strippers, were more fantastic productions, flowering visions that jolted me awake and were elaborated in rapid scribbles over three or four pages. One I remember described the huge winged creatures (whose name I have forgotten), tentacled like octopi, who raided our dimension to suck the life force from humans through their eyes; the people one encountered on the street, most of us in fact, were the remains of their depredations. Where to send such a poem but to the Antipodes, as far from home as was geographically possible? But *Poetry Australia,* though they had previously accepted a short poem synchronizing the flowering of a hawthorn tree with the life of Heinrich Himmler, returned this one without comment.

completely arbitrary. Unaccountable, they do with you what they will.

That was certainly the case on the playground, which seemed to me an extreme classroom, its rules warped to multiply thrill and terror. Behind the school stretched a plain, vast to my eyes, of patches of stubbled grass surrounded by hard, pale dirt pounded flat by hordes of running feet. "They're coming!" the cry would go up, as we played Red Rover or British Bulldog in the grassiest, softest-for-falling area. Across the plain, as we stood gaping, a dust cloud roiled toward us, like the dust of a prairie stampede. We milled together, like zebras or antelopes before a lion attack, and then, just as in the animal documentaries, scattered in all directions as the bullies converged to pick off their targets. I was seldom damaged, except collaterally, when a whole storm of bodies crashed together. I was middle-sized, with a middle expression: neither big nor small, neither bold nor visibly afraid; not ostentatiously "different" enough to constitute a challenge or an obvious victim.

The most different person was never attacked. Neither by the bullies nor by their whimpering victims, who often, in the aftermath of an assault, turned on one another. Everyone understood on an intuitive level that extreme difference breeds strange powers and entanglements, magical complications that transcend the laws of physical force. To cross far enough over was to be inviolate, though at the price of utter isolation.

Paul Tamburlaine. What do I really remember of him? I don't want to stitch him together with imaginary threads. Watery, rather expressionless eyes, pale grey infused with jots of blue. A wide gash of delight, which split his face at odd moments, for no apparent cause, exposing a wet red mouth and large, crooked teeth. Thin arms with large, clumsy fingers. A slow, lurching walk. I remember more of him than I thought; he is wobbling into view. His most obvious feature, so obvious that after a while you seldom noticed it, was his greatly enlarged head. Bulbed at the forehead and behind, it suggested the shape of a light bulb, with his face in the narrowing part. His swollen head, still swelling, was the result of a fall from a tree when he was younger; that was the story that circulated.

Paul sat or stood at the perimeter of things. He seemed content there. His desk was at the back of the grade two classroom, moved a few inches closer to the corner so the teacher could squeeze by when checking the other students' work. Colouring with a box of crayons is how I remember him spending his time. He was larger than a grade two, and looked older by a year or more; grade two may have been only a convenient spot to keep him, or perhaps it was the place he'd been when his accident had arrested his progress. Outside, he stood by the sidewalk at the far edge of the playground, scratching, with a stick he'd found, things in the dirt. He watched us at times, that sudden grin baring the lurid mouth, but usually just stood with his head down. He could talk, and reply to simple questions, but he rarely spoke or was spoken to. His voice was unnervingly high-pitched; there was a screeching note, a hint of frenzy, in it even when he was speaking quietly. From time to time a new student would invite him to join a game. By the firm shake of his head, No, it seemed he had been told not to play, perhaps because of further risk to his head. He was often away from school, for medical appointments we were told.

For a time, Paul was my closest companion. Not at school, where such a blurring of categories would have subjected me (not Paul) to violent censure. Paul seemed to understand this, grinning my way only slightly more often than before. But his house was on the way to mine, and I often went to his yard after school. My parents, if they noticed this at all (they were busy, their fifth child on the way, and I was already an expert evader), might have construed it as a way of adjusting to a new milieu. Paul's mother was more concerned, parting the front curtains every few minutes to peer out at us. Calling sometimes, "Pa-ul?", whereupon he would go inside for a time and then rejoin me.

Our minutes together—or hours, since they seemed timeless—were some of the most peaceful I have ever spent, and even to think of that short autumn launches me on a wave of nostalgia. Curiously, since those intervals were almost entirely wordless, it is most often while writing that I approach the same borderland of poised still-ness, a kind of scooped-out expectancy, that makes me think of Paul. Though his mother may have wondered at my motives in befriending her brain-damaged boy, I was simply drawn to him. I liked his otherness and his quiet occupations. I liked his silences and the occasional grating cries that punctuated them. They meshed with my own inner cycles of reverie and happy accident, and many years later they would return to me as early prefigurations of my notion of sanity as a perpetual guerrilla action, raids on incoherence.

A big pine tree dominated Paul's front yard (I assumed, without any evidence, that it was the tree he had fallen from), its bushy, sweeping branches shading half the lot, creating a cozy, grassless circle of needles and dirt around its base. Paul would be in there, among the sun-and-shadow patterns, drawing marks with a stick. I stood nearby, watching him. The things he drew were always the same. Or they were meant to be, I think, since his physical awkwardness and the resistance of the dirt sometimes skewed them out of shape. They were the same symbols he drew everywhere. (Except in class, where he crayoned clumsier versions of the generic landscape we had all learned: sun, cloud, grass, tree, house.) He drew a stroke across from left to right, then a longer stroke down starting at the first stroke's right end. To the right of this first figure, he scratched a circle, concentrating to do so without lifting his stick. Of the three strokes, the circle was hardest, often wobbling out of course around a stone or a hard clump of dirt. The resulting shapes looked roughly like the number 70. But only roughly, since the angles of the first two strokes and the size and position of the circle were so changeable. They could also look like the number 10, since Paul sometimes dug his stick in hard, grinding it back and forth, at the bottom of the second stroke.

I'm thinking of Paul's marks as numbers now, to describe them. I don't remember doing so at the time. They were just Paul's marks. They were his voice really, more focused and more personal than those strangled yelps he emitted. Milling with the other students at recess, before or after the bullies had attacked, I would look across the schoolyard plain and see Paul at the edge, head down, drawing with his stick. It was comforting to know what he was drawing, as if I was *there* while standing *here,* and especially to know that he *was drawing.* The tasks of school had already thrown the rest of us into an oppositional sloth, an ostentatious indolence to counter our enforced diligence, but Paul had escaped this teeter-totter of rote and recoil. He was always busy in his own world, etching his intentions upon it, like the much younger child the rest of us had already left far behind.

Fights between bullies, which happened once or twice a week, took place against a red brick wall at the back of the school. I almost said *were staged,* since this wall of bare, chipped brick, its putty darkened with graffiti the janitors couldn't scrub off, was the perfect backdrop to the spectacle we watched from a crowded semicircle. The combatants were sealed in between the brick and the packed onlookers. Usually it was two of the minor bullies fighting, perhaps to settle a dispute or to advance their standing; we knew nothing of the inner workings of the gang. Every so often, though, as the climax of a cycle in which the minor fights were epicycles, the two main bullies fought, a treat that was announced in excited whispers for days beforehand. Moose and Hackney exchanged places regularly as leader of the bullies. The fights were real—flying blood and snot and curses, smashing fists and feet—but their prize seemed more symbolic than real. The one who was not leader afterward was his close subordinate, almost equal in power of command, and was alone in being immune from the leader who had just narrowly defeated him and whom he would soon narrowly defeat…an endless cycle. Endless, at least, until they turned sixteen and could finally leave grade eight, where they had strutted and fought for years. Moose and Hackney. They were like contrasting types in a western, interchangeable as villain and hero but visually distinct for the viewer's convenience. Moose short and broad and blond, Hackney tall and skinny and black-haired. Both wore nosepicker cowboy boots, for clicking and kicking.

Standing among the youngest students at the rear, I would look away from the din—from the back it was mostly an auditory event, a tumult of screams and thuds and the special crunches that brought deep-bellied groans of pain and appreciation—and see Paul over at the edge of the

playground, his stick dangling from his hand, watching
us. Or watching the place where the noise came from; his
posture seemed attentive but not curious. His position
looked so peaceful. Occasionally a car passed behind him,
the only motion on those streets of silent bungalows. At
some point—I don't know when it started or in what
terms I conceived of it then—I understood that Paul was
the most powerful person in our school. I don't know if it
was a thought, I don't know if I had thoughts then. Years
later, in my sci-fi phase, I might have imagined Paul direct-
ing the proceedings, all of us, with thought-beams. It might
unfold that way in a *Twilight Zone* episode, the nobody on
the margins who was actually the alien in command. But
this was far less conceptualized; it felt like simple recognition. It was also a longing, an intuitive attraction to Paul's
weird and singular privilege. Bullies traded places; Paul
kept his. No one bothered him: not students, not teachers, not even the principal. Bullies, I noticed, even
Moose and Hackney, slouched past him as if he wasn't
there, feigning obliviousness instead of inflicting it.
Sometimes when they passed Paul I caught a confused—
almost a *lost*—look on their faces. Those looks
disconcerted and hinted at something thrilling. The
leaders' power fell away from them in an arena in which
it had no meaning. I couldn't begin to understand any of
this. At that age all motion, all awareness, was merely
magnetic: I never decided to move, only felt myself moving, creeping toward some things, inching away from

others. Things and people approaching or receding told me I was moving.

Whatever this dawning revelation was, about Paul and about power at the margins, I knew enough not to tell it to anyone. I kept it close and secret, something to nourish and prove my allegiance to, much as a sorcerer might add each new herb he collects to a bundle tied in a leather purse that he hangs inside his clothes, next to the private heat of his body.

Sometime that fall, Paul left our school. He may have lived at home for a time without going to any school, because I have a few memories of passing his house and seeing him standing near the pine tree with his stick. I didn't stop anymore, and he didn't raise his large, pale face as if he expected me to. By then, by processes occult to me, I had been absorbed into the normal life of school, where I was beginning to excel.

Paul was gone by that late autumn day when a great adult excitement communicated itself to us and we were let out of school early. Everything seemed chaotically off, festively traumatic, like a daytime Halloween. Kids milled around in unusual knots, a goofy boy with red hair ran around shouting, "The King's dead! The King's dead!" We waited for our mothers to pick us up, even those of us who normally walked home. Some of the mothers in the station wagons were crying; two of them got out and hugged each other. Paul is nowhere in the scene, but some essence of him clings to what I recall, blended with my activities as if I had absorbed him, as if we were now one person. Lying on the living room floor for the next two days in front of the television which was never off. My parents smoking and talking in low voices. They talked mostly about the King with the huge head, and the little man who had killed him. By now, of course, I knew the facts behind the redhead's leering cry, "The King's dead! The King's dead!" But his version, like a peasant's shout in a fairy tale, still seemed truest. Black horses, one riderless; cannons; the avenue thronged with weeping subjects; the beautiful, veiled Queen: what were these but the trappings of a dead King? Lying on the floor with my paper and crayons below the hanging smoke, I drew a version of Moose and Hackney, but the colours and proportions were wrong. Plus, I couldn't draw a gun. Then, at some point, I got another idea from the pictures on TV. The bullets that blew apart the King's huge head came from high up in a corner, so far away that the little man in the window with his gun couldn't be seen, a TV man had to draw a circle around the spot. And then, when the little man himself got killed, again it was by an arm coming out of the corner. My first three months at Chedoke Public School, and Paul in particular, had prepared me to understand this. The adults were always talking about the man in the middle, but all the real power was over at the side, almost out of sight, in the corner. That power could blow a King's head off, snatch a prisoner from the arms of big policemen. From time to time I glanced up warily at my parents. They seemed utterly absorbed in the TV accounts, never hinting by a look or comment that they doubted them. Didn't they know the power was at the margins? Or did they know and pretend not to? Both possibilities unnerved me, and I ducked back down into my drawing, shrinking my world to paper and coloured wax.

Finally, I found a way to hint at what I was seeing. It didn't convey my understanding, but it gestured toward it. I filled in some patches of grey and white, mixed with bits of beige, in the middle of my paper. It looked like a muddle of ragged clouds, a jigsaw fog. Then, over in one corner, I put a long black bar, with a short red bar coming out of it—like a figure in black with a red hand, or gun. I made the red and black lines as strong as I could, pressing over them again and again until they gleamed darkly. I kept redoing the drawing, changing the sizes and configurations of the centre shapes and the corner figure, trying the latter in different corners, for instance. I could never get it quite right, but I liked the general effect. It was the kind of thing I wanted to do more of.

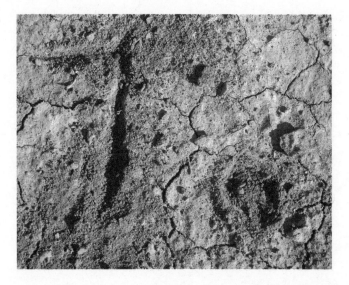

Next I became aware of my watch malfunctioning. By "next" I mean not just the next step in a sequence but the next signal from the same transmission. If you are making your way through a forest, the way may be easy or hard, but neither case is like coming upon a cleared path laid out in a direction that beckons you. And if, a little later, the path breaks down, petering out on rock or becoming choked with deadfall, then pressing forward in what you construe to be the same direction is nothing like the way opening suddenly underfoot and up ahead so that you find yourself on the clear and shining trail again.

My watch was breaking down. But not all at once and not completely, which for a while prevented me from repairing it. I would notice it was running two minutes slow. An hour later, it had lost another minute. Okay, I thought. I set it to the radio and checked it six hours later. Perfect time. Two days later, still perfect. A bit of dust inside the works? The next morning it would be five minutes behind (it was never fast). This was a couple of weeks after the Schama/Picasso overlay, and I took it to be part of the same dance with time. It was an instinct that kicked in about certain symmetries coalescing, which led me to issue myself mental reminders: *Take note. Stay alert.* ("Stay frosty," a movie Marine would have growled.) I started keeping the watch in my pocket, it was less unnerving than having its uncertainty on my wrist. I asked people what time it was. People I was meeting. Then strangers. Most replied politely, but a few gave me sharp looks, this beggar bumming time instead of coins. The results stayed variable. Right on the dot. A minute off. (It was never fast.) A half-hour behind—now we're talking! Dead accurate for the next four days. Always this nagging little drama, this stutter-step from a Beckett notebook: breaking (or?), must break (or?), stagger on (. . . or?). When I finally took it to a jeweller in a mall, it wasn't because the watch had definitely died (though what would that mean? it had lain dormant for hours —why not a year?) but because I was sick of the space it was occupying in my mind.

I stared at the glitter of expensive watches under glass while the sales clerk finished with another customer. She frowned when I stated my problem. One of those natural young Mediterranean beauties—big dark eyes, chestnut hair, she would have stopped your heart drying her hair after a shower—who had smothered herself in makeup and floral scent. She limped in her stiletto heels.

She came back and told me that the battery was fine. I was prepared for that possibility, though still a little surprised. A cleaning? I inquired. No—she gestured at the door behind her; I saw a little man, bald, bent over a cluttered desk—he said it was fine, no dust. I stood there stunned, my not-dead watch in my hand. The hand she laid on the counter had inch-long, curving nails the colour of whiteout. Did I want to buy a strap?

All of the transferring between wrist and pocket had cracked the old strap almost through. Her father—some shared liquidity in the eyes when he turned to her— attached a new leather strap to my failing but not failed watch. For a few days it kept perfect time.

. . .

The laws of breakdown. Its code. Which you must on no account violate if the breakdown is to be yours (and of what use would another's be?). Perpetual vigilance is required, the paradox of rigour amid crack-up (which is in fact no paradox but a precondition). What you don't want above all, the worst betrayal—of the process, of yourself, of life even—is a botched breakdown. One of those tape-and-glue stumble-ons that can simulate recovery, functionality, can even, with a protraction that a Torquemada might flinch from inflicting, extend themselves into a slow-motion suicide lasting seventy years or more, "sadly missed."

No. (That much you know.)

Eventually the watch will stop. Or you will smash it: that seems daily more likely. Beyond a stopped watch will be . . . no time or new time. But not fractured time. Not these splintered and dissolving minutes.

Beware of watch repairmen. Tinkerers. Parts-replacers. *Let the watch break.*

(And yet no way to tell, from the first slip-slidings out of time—or the first noticing of them, for who remarks on a few dropped seconds?—how long it will take a watch to break. Days? Weeks? Years? More time than a lifetime affords?

To smash, crash, stop. And become . . . time-less, bare-wristed? Or tell time true, anew?

Or be tinkered back to passability? Fiddled with and spit-shined by the old, bald man?

No way, ultimately, to know.)

. . .

During my first year at university I dwelt in a kind of twilight state that I called a waking dream. This state was so strange that I assumed it could not last long. Yet it would last another four years and lead, not to the death or awakening I expected, but only to long-term hospitalization. It wasn't like a dream, not really, but it wasn't waking life either. Perhaps "waking dream" is really the best way to describe it. Precisely imprecise.

I had trouble telling the time. Clocks and watches told me one thing, but my eyes told me another. It might be noon, but the colours were leaching from things and a grainy veil was drawing over them (I rubbed my eyes until they bruised)—as if the world had been sketched with almost-dry markers, then photographed out of focus, while a machine blew in fine grey specks, sand or soot, that floated and sank—I piled up the scenarios that could conjure the faded, sleazy dregs I was seeing. And it went the other way too. Out walking at 3 a.m.—I took these epic tramps to try to exhaust myself into sleep—I'd pass another nighthawk and see, in a scream of light, a face or part of a face. A nose, a chin, a forehead. Autopsy-sheer, pinned under ferocious white. I stopped and gaped, startling the other into a jog, glancing back over their shoulder. And I looked about for the street light or passing car responsible for the light-burst. But there was nothing. I was standing on a darkened street, the footsteps *pat-pat-pat*ting away.

I tested my eyes in the mirror. Even if nothing was seriously wrong with them, maybe I'd developed a tic of staring and squinting; my own lashes could be that mesh I seemed to be peering through. It was only a slim, desperate hope, which I didn't really believe. Otherwise, why did my guts knot as I approached the medicine cabinet's mirrored door? I'd learned to wash and brush and shave without looking up except in slivers, spotting the part I needed to clip or dry. Now I looked straight on, eyes open. Black. That was the first thing I noticed. My eyes couldn't be called brown, even dark brown, anymore. Black buttons, with a plasticky gleam; sunk in grey, puffy folds. But they were open. And still the light from the forty-watt bulb flickered up and down, like someone twiddling a dimmer switch. The face in the glass frightened me. It was a mask behind which great error was occurring. Sometimes I thought of the error as evil. There was a moral dimension—that somehow I had chosen this—that I couldn't shake.

For long hours, twisted in the sheets of my rooming house bed, I lay in a swamp void of volition, twitching my hand or foot to be sure I wasn't actually paralyzed. I had left my parents' house abruptly, taking my shaving kit and a few clothes. Not just to be free of them—I was eighteen— but to find a quiet place where *it* could happen. I felt a shame about what was coming and for as long as possible I wanted it to happen out of sight. Some animal instinct for the time for crawling away. I never lost the sense, even when the turns got frankly terrible, that there was a knowingness, some cruel wisdom, guiding the process. Something ancient knew all this, perhaps had coded it through millennia, and had procedures even in the midst of chaos. That kind of thinking irritated the interviewers later. They wanted me to say it was all bad, all symptom. Pathology to be chucked while I steered toward health. And I couldn't, quite. It wasn't stubbornness, nor courage— I was terrified. Sickened and disgusted and mesmerized by dread. But to give up all glimmers of knowing, of sensing landmarks and direction—where, what would that leave you? Even in the blackest mangrove swamp, sunk there on a moonless midnight, you had to claw-squelch-flail-inch toward something—you couldn't just *hang* there. Why couldn't they see that? I'd stare at them (*confrontational* they must have noted), really trying to figure it. But that was all up ahead.

For now, I was nothing but symptoms. Such a profusion of them it paints too orderly a picture to give these examples. Symptoms like an anthill, boot-strewn: cognitive, affective, behavioural. Physical, metabolic: hair texture, skin tone, digestion—all wacko. A total stone.[3]

Except that I didn't use the word *symptoms*, not to myself. It wasn't my word. It was something more like travel, a process unfolding. And so close I didn't need to name it. A secret knowledge that I came to call a pregnancy. A pact. An interior pact of tremendous vitality. Vitality

---

3 Doing drugs brought temporary relief and then a longer sadness. Acid, mescaline, grass, hash, speed: they gave reasons for things to be altered, though even so, the alterations were milder. And others to be altered with—though they would not be altered in the morning. Would just be grumbling about coming down, reaching for the Cheerios. People naturally assumed I was doing more drugs—at a glance I might have passed for a stoner—but the small relief wasn't worth the loneliness, and I was doing them less all the time.

and risk, a doomed cellular glamour. Soon, I'd think. We're almost there. It's coming, not much longer. It'll be bad, really atrocious . . . but then it will be over.

All these steady mantras to get me past the moments.

There were gaps. Blink-outs. There must have been, because I'd find myself somewhere—in a park, on a street, in a room—with no memories of having got there. I'd think back, hard. Like a math problem. Standing in a park. Winter. Snow, stars. Back . . . the coffee shop. Low light but not dark, more like dusk. Hours ago, then. An hour or two at least. What else? Try! Nothing. A blank spool between then and now. I wasn't there. Not in my own memory. Where was I, then? (Where am I?)[4]

I didn't *invent* The Autopilot, I said testily, one of the rare times my voice rose, in one of the offices later. (The pen scratching its evidence, the thin lips pursing.) I simply gave a name, an obvious name, to something that needed one. Someone—Something—was moving me from A to B. A phenomenon. It matters, so you name it. Right?

When it wasn't rinsed by radiance—the Illuminations were becoming less frequent, something settling down, locking in—the world looked wretchedly dirty. The Ugly

---

4 Absence seizures, more common in childhood and caused by a mild impairment of the interaction of the thalamus with cortical grey matter, produce a momentary clouding of consciousness, as when one stares at a bonfire or blank wall. They correlate with brief but abnormal patterns of neuronal firing that may originate in the intralaminar nuclei of the thalamus. But departures on the time scale I experienced them—hours, occasionally days—would have to be called fugue states, I think. Even a series of absence seizures over a short time would presumably leave some fragments of recollection between them.

was everywhere. Grime spattering the window glass. Streaking the walls, the floor, the ceiling. Hanging in filthy webs, putrid, decaying streamers. Everything was grime. I was grime.

I'd forget to eat for two days and then shovel down a pot of Kraft Dinner at 4 a.m., gobbling it over the filthy stove. Wander along wondering seriously how I could be feeling so cold, whatever happened to the warm blood of youth, and could I really have lost all muscle tone that fast, then notice, like a sign posted in the corner of my eye, an icicle, and then another notice, my red T-shirt, bare arm. February, I'd remember. And sometimes burst out laughing at such times, not always crazily, sometimes just a really warm chuckle at how goofy it was all getting. Oh, Grandma, what a Big Sicko you've become!

(The marvel of it, the astonishment even now, is how closely, and for how long, you can skirt an edge before going over it. So strange, yet familiar: it is the suave enticement of seduction, of grooming. The cruellest thing symptoms do is make you love them.)

I knew enough to steer clear of people. I moved through McMaster's campus like a ghost through a fleshed town. I was especially afraid of meeting former classmates, afraid they'd try to talk to the smart, affable guy they'd known and we'd both feel weird, so I found a lot of back alleys and unused stairwells, kept my head down. There was a system inside things, I found, a sort of parallel architecture that allowed you to stay invisible and still get where you needed to be, ghost routes so dependable they seemed as planned as washrooms. I assumed I looked awful, a real ratbag out of Dostoevsky's notebooks, and was shocked sometimes when a normal-looking person gave me a smile or chatted to me in the coffee line. Was it all invisible? I couldn't credit it for long. Especially, I worried about the two dimensions meeting, inner and outer, ghost and flesh—I imagined something like the matter/antimatter cataclysm in *Star Trek*. Even a slight leak could cause a lot of local damage.

I think it may have happened once. There was a girl— intelligent-looking, with kind eyes and a large hooked nose—I kept running into. I'd catch her giving me these sad, strangely pointed looks; searching glances, as if she knew me partway and couldn't figure out another part. I started seeing her more and more, and the looks became more intense. Meeting them with what I thought was a neutral expression, I would see her jerk away suddenly, as if she had burst into tears or was about to. This went on for a time, the tension of our meetings mounting, and then—I don't think I called them transmissions yet—some pictures came into my head. She is looking up at me, we are dancing a slow dance, just circling slowly in a crowd, she is smiling, her eyes warm, and I feel the dampness of her blouse where I am holding her. Her name flits near, like a word on a passing radio, and then is gone. And then her face again below me, in shadow, in a bed, she is holding the covers over her breasts and I see the white glow of her chest, a dark flush at the base of her throat. She is frowning slightly. She looks puzzled, angry. She is trying to figure out something that is hurting her. Where am I? I must be beside the bed, from the angle.

That was all. But now that I'd seen them, the pictures stayed, strong and consistent. And they made a kind of story that went with her stricken, resentful looks. Had we really met at a pub, gone to her room? And then I'd forgotten the night, forgotten her? How awful. There was real damage here. The gaps so complete, anything between them possible. And no way to tell her, no way to explain. She'd have to be with me, all the way in, sharing our lives. And I was far beyond that (or before it, below it, really). It did flicker in my mind, a flitting hope like her vanished name, which for a short time made our chance meetings even more charged. Stay away from people, I told myself. And then I stopped seeing her, we never met again. I still think about her occasionally, wonder what really happened. Where she is now and what she made of it then. The pictures separate and distinct as ever. Still no name.

I knew I had to quit university, had to make it official, but I still dropped in to classes once in a while, read the odd page. Showed up for exams, handed in papers—I must've, because my transcript lists low Bs, the subjects passed. I don't know whether that proves how little arts programs

were asking even then, in the mid-1970s, or how ripped my
academic muscles had become by senior high school, so
that I could coast for a long time while they turned to flab—
both, probably. I recall almost none of it. If interrogators
put a gun to my head and ordered me to write down everything I remember from my first two years of university, *only
true memories no lying,* I couldn't fill a page. Not with school
memories: classrooms, teachers, other students. Things I
read. They didn't happen. Not if memories equal events,
they didn't. The coffee I just made happened more.

One note on the page. No date. A philosophy class. The
grad student, a tall beard, is trying to impress us with first-
year conundrums. The tree in the forest. How do I know I
know? When he gets to the one about the Chinese philoso-
pher who dreamed he was a butterfly, and ever afterward
wondered which he really was, man dreaming butterfly or
butterfly dreaming man, the students chuckle dryly. That
rouses me. I say something to the effect that obviously
they'd never had a sufficiently compelling dream. No other
storyline had tempted them. Something like that; probably
in a rusty, too-loud voice, since the heads jerking around is
a sharp image. I'm slouched in a back corner, the Raskol-
nikov seat reserved for the shitbird who drifts in once a
month to sneer at the proceedings. The beard shoots me a
look of appreciation: a baby Nietzsche I can nourish? Then
a cold remorse and shame washes over me, like a cup of ice
water I'd tried to dash in people's faces and it had blown
back in my own. I feel awake for an instant, really awake,

and think, What are you doing here? You don't belong with any of this. Get out, get out, get out. You're way past due.

The dream of Liesl Annerkant. 1970. Grade ten. I look back on it as the zenith of my school career, because even though my marks climbed higher in the next two years, some dispersal must have started too, it seems likely, for it all to fall away so quickly in grade thirteen. Yet I know nothing of the timing, and only a little about the process. But a view of something that you know is about to break does not look solid; some awareness of the breakage seeps back into the earlier frames; you have to snip out quite a bit of infected film to get a shot that feels reasonably solid. And so, by subtraction, I arrive at the solidity of grade ten: a compact coherence, packing my bones and spirit tight together. A real good boy, young man. I have two close friends, we play Risk and penny poker. Sip whiskey, trade jokes and insults and sex fantasies. I join the euchre tournament in the cafeteria. Play road hockey behind the Salvation Army. I make the football team, not first string, but I get in a few plays. None of my marks is under 80 and I am getting 98 in Math.

Liesl Annerkant, two rows over, is getting 100. She hasn't made an error yet. Not one decimal out of place. Her perfect string creates a delicious tension in the room: Can she keep it up? Mr Brieve, who has a sense of drama, draws out the moment when he hands back tests, approaching her desk with a blank face that kills us, not grave, not anything. We *squirm*. And then he slams down her paper, slaps it like a high-five on wood, face up with the three big, perfect numerals circled in red. And a cheer goes up, it breaks out of us: "An' she can!" The best we have been able to do with her awkward German name. And Liesl, not shy but not a gloater, lowers her head, peers with a frown like factoring at her own perfection, there is nowhere else to look, while two spots of rose glow on the back of her long, slender neck. She is beautiful. I can't introduce flaws just to keep the picture interesting. Full-breasted, slim-waisted, long-legged; with a stern, straight nose like Athena in our myths book—and wheat-blond hair, long and centre-parted. And nice: not overly friendly, but always patient if someone needs help, smiling when you pass in the hall. Just an achingly good, achingly gifted girl. A perfect girl. Why shy from the word?

And, curiously, nobody seemed to have it in for her. Not even the other girls. All the nastiness that ten years had taught us, all the endless, petty battlegrounds that were school—something, her sheerness it must have been, lifted Liesl clear of all that. You didn't hear catty remarks about her. You didn't hear horny ones either. She was better-looking by far than any of the girls we lusted grimly after, degrading them in our convoluted jokes—but she didn't enter our minds that way. It would have been like mating with another species. It must have been a kind of loneliness for her. This sphere of spotless admiration and goodwill that she floated in, untouched and untouchable.

I dreamed of her one night. It was the most remarkable dream I'd ever had—its singularity strikes me to this day—and not only was I a long time getting over it, but it seemed to shift me on my axis permanently, sticking me at a slightly altered angle into the world. The dream itself is simplicity to tell. Its seamless simplicity is what made it so haunting.

In the dream, Liesl and I live a long, rich life together. We share a small house. There are no children. My work is bureaucratic, some kind of applied science in an office, but Liesl's gifts are still leading her to the heights. She is a star of pure mathematics, and a highlight of our days is her describing some exciting new aspect of her research as we make dinner together. Both of us frowning, and then laughing helplessly, as I try, and try, and finally fail, to follow some obscure point. Such talk! Of a depth and richness, a variety and constancy, that I have never imagined in my waking life. Pet jokes, gossip, even boredom, stale topics that bring aggravation, sharp digs. The whole shared life in words. Sex is there, delicious interludes, but even it is secondary to this consuming conversation. The dream's resources are those of a master of exhaustive realism. No quirk or oddity ever feels imposed upon a scene, but none is overlooked if it is intrinsic to it—everywhere is the enthralling wealth, the minutely observed texture of the life we have together. If that life is so much richer than any I have known, charged with a shining meaning, it is because I am finally *in* life, draped in its fabric, attentive to every thread. I was conscious of this in the dream, without being conscious I was dreaming. This, *this,* is it, I thought, with gasping gratitude. *This* is how you do it. This is how it *is.* There is pain. Of course there is. Nothing is missing. Illness, heartache, disappointment. Betrayal, bitter words, tears. We even age convincingly, in tandem but differently: my hair thinning but staying mostly dark, Liesl's going steely grey; me growing paunchy, soft, while she becomes leaner, almost gaunt. I comfort her in those moments, more numerous as she ages, when her confidence falters ("An' she *can!*"). She comforts me wordlessly, with a look or touch.

Always, uniting all the multitudinous scenes, is our talk, the guiding current, this river of achieved communion...murmuring in the bedroom's dusk, rippling and splashing in the yellow kitchen after work, pooling in wide, silent bays...carrying, in all its sparkling surfaces and turbid depths, our whole vast history onward toward something unseen...

I awake and lie very still in my bed. For a few minutes there is nothing but a sense of suspension and well-being, a warm bath of utter contentment. Then, in tiny increments, I begin to be aware of other feelings, doubts and confusions like small stinging insects that are dragging me back into another, lesser reality. The dream is so alien to my real circumstances, my life as a fifteen-year-old boy. Which, in the wake of the dream, does not seem more real, only more threadbare. Like emerging from a long opera to hear some of the same tunes played on a kazoo. My rocket ship bank on the bookcase, a gift from an aunt some years ago. The sounds of my parents downstairs. It is heartbreaking to be dropped back into this, cruel for the dream even to have shown itself to me.[5]

Questions help a bit. I can cling to the dream aura a bit longer through them, prevent it from receding too fast. How had a lifetime, two long lives, been compressed into one night? The best answer I can come up with (the reality of the dream being too absolute to question) is that I am living that life in a parallel universe, where none of the same laws, including those of time, apply. (The aesthetic answer I would hazard now, that the dream director stuffed a scene so convincingly that it summoned others in its train, did not occur to me then.) Perhaps I can return to it. Do my time in this one, quietly, trying not to jar the portal, and slip back through. Perhaps even tonight.

Rain that had frozen during the night had coated the trees outside my window with ice, the trunks inside clear columns, the twig ends hanging in clear, glassy bells. Light pulsed back from the crust, like clear shellac, on the snow. Liesl was out there somewhere, dressing in her room. I didn't know where she lived. Was it possible she

---

5 To this day I wonder whether the dream was a valediction to normalcy, to fitting myself satisfactorily inside the world with other people—or a prediction, a reassurance from some deep source, that that *was* my home and, after straying very far, I would return to it. A goodbye to, or a promise of eventual, sanity?

had not experienced the same dream? No. Telepathy at a minimum was what we'd shared.

Downstairs, my parents were eating their toast, sipping their black coffee. Not talking, thankfully. I got my cereal bowl and took my place. Holding on to the dream's spell was a fragile effort, more precarious by the minute. But their silence and small noises, clinks and scrapings— these were suspicious. They brought back doubts I had had at the time of Paul Tamburlaine. The dream's momentousness so filled me that I knew I was changed utterly. Could they really be oblivious of that, or were they pretending to be? Were they actors or automatons?

I crossed an open field before I reached the streets around the school. The freezing had formed a perfect crust that allowed me, with delicate steps, to walk on top of it, on a film between ground and sky, above a piled fleecy whiteness that my occasional plunges through let me wallow in. In hollows where the water had pooled and the ice was thicker, I took three quick steps and went gliding, sailing, finally quite weightless. The air was still after the storm. Still as the inside of a bell.

In math class Liesl was bent over her work as usual, giving no sign. The thin mockery of school life had prepared me for the moment, easing, in what seemed a self-betrayal, the pricklings in my stomach. Getting back was going to be more difficult, I saw, more occult. I would have to be vigilant. Who knew when I would return to the Reality Dream? (Never, as it turned out, at least not in the same form.) In the meantime, like a desolated scientist, I noted the differences between the dream and so-called waking life, to the radical disparagement of the latter. The discontinuity of time, moments like beads without a thread to join them. The confusion, the lack of purpose. Like a bunch of lolling, empty-headed actors who, out of sheer boredom, sometimes improvise inept little skits, then fall to dozing again. The adequate, undramatic light. The tinniness. The threadbareness.[6] I tried to summon a knowing cynicism, but when I thought of the dream, I felt sick at heart. It faded only very slowly, leaving a residue of longing and bitterness that was acute for a time and fitful for a long time after that.

Curiously, I began to take less notice of Liesl. I had known—would know?—her somewhere else, but things were different here. As a notion that she was a figure

---

6 The dream as 600-thread-count sheet, which, while not more real than a cheap sheet, may convince one fortunate enough to sleep on it that this, *really*, is what sleeping is. It wasn't that life in the dream was better than my life awake; it may have been worse. Petty disagreements, even tearful and cruel quarrels, were frequent in it, as were episodes of sickness and loss, wild, barren grief. What made the dream so heartbreaking was its vivid continuity, its sense of a life solid and dimensional—slice into it from any angle and you would find the same stuff, the same rich meat. My sorrow, which amazed me scarcely less at the time than my dream, may have been my intuition, as yet inarticulable, of the chasm opening up between that meaty seamlessness and the ghostly discontinuity, luminous fragments with dead air like test pattern static between them, that life would soon become and must already have begun becoming. The dream was a cry for wholeness, for solid earth from one sinking into quicksand. It was a sumptuous film created to counter a dread of scissored frames.

from the future crept into me and took silent hold, her present self, a premonitory figment only, dissolved.

Over the next two years I sank, half deliberately, into a dreamy inwardness, a lush romanticism that kept an active gregariousness around it like a hard shell protecting a creamy yolk. Piano playing was the natural art form to express this. For years I had practised my Conservatory lessons diligently, but now I poured myself into music, composing song after song. Having artistic "leanings" but no proper medium was a problem that had nagged me for a long time,[7] but I felt I'd solved it now. Visual arts had been my first love, but past the colouring stage, my utter lack of talent was prohibitive. With music I had at least manual dexterity, good rhythm, a so-so ear. I thought that with the engine of a blinding work ethic I could whip these raw materials into something. I wrote sugary melodies over minor descending chords, often with an arpeggiated introduction that showed off my speed. My pride in them was dampened occasionally by a suspicion that they

---

7 Facility at mimicry and a persevering work ethic hid for a long time the nature of any individual talent I might possess, and despite my best efforts they still obscure this, especially when I am working too slowly. Working at top speed, for all the problems it causes, is a way of keeping my instincts out ahead of the various learned programs that stand ready to check and supplant them. Having abilities that were slightly above average in several areas made it difficult to find a true direction. Over and over I found myself too proficient to give up, but not talented enough to gain real confidence. In a road hockey game, if twelve boys were available for teams, I would be picked fourth or fifth—too early to squelch hope and too late to firmly nourish it. Likewise, many expressed pleasure in my songs, a few marvelled at them; no one asked to hear them.

resembled other songs; greater musicality would have recognized their progenitors instantly. When I presented one of these songs to my first girlfriend, inscribed in black pen on musical notepaper and played on an accompanying cassette, its title an anagram of our names, she was moved to tears. My adoration of her intensified, mingled with, inextricable from, a sense of my own omnipotence. Later, after playing it dozens of times to myself, I felt a bit disdainful of us both. Aside from the occasional oddity, such as a mournful and repetitive elegy for Charlotte Corday, the guillotined assassin of Jean-Paul Marat, my other kind of song was pure noise, waves of crashing discords, that I found particularly inspired and strangely relaxing. No one else enjoyed these, though, and, worse, some people thought I was joking when I played them. When the house was empty, I felt a strange exultation, a kind of energizing alarm, in sending my sugar pops and my clashing tumults billowing in alternating waves that finally cancelled out in exhaustion and a surfeited peace.[8]

---

8 The musical limitations that prevented me from recognizing my pop songs as derivative, and hearing that my noise was just loud bad harmonies, were typified by a mistake I made in mathematics, sister of music. Mr Brieve told us of the unsolved problem of trisecting an angle, a long-standing math conundrum with a prize offered for its solution. With two friends I worked all one heady night solving the problem. We had the solution ready on a side blackboard the next morning. Mr Brieve, with a smile he quickly suppressed, pointed out that although we had done good work in trisecting the line we had drawn between the angle's two rays, we had forgotten that an angle comprised, not a line, but the degrees in a circle's arc. As the leader of the group, I was most embarrassed. I might be getting 98, but in mathematical terms I had just demonstrated a tin ear. Liesl, passing by on her way to her seat, smiled good-naturedly. Brilliant as she was, she was not even a snob.

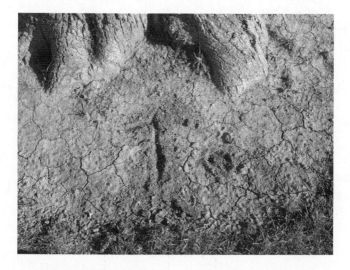

The conference room. (1978?) The murk parts and I see
knees, in blue jeans, almost touching larger knees in
brown cords. Fog slides, the hole widens.

Slowly, I raise my eyes. Silver sun buckle. Oh, oh. Big
gut and chest, in blue checks. Now the face. A huge one,
scowling. Walrus moustache, long blond shag. Oh, oh, oh.

Thirty-eight, he says. The name already past, I missed
it. He'd been a steelworker, a millwright. Is now a doctor.
A psychiatry resident. It is all barked out in a deep

almost-growl. In my face, like I bumped him in a prison yard. Do I understand?

I nod, careful to blank my eyes. No matter how much danger I've kept time with, he is taking me further back, back to first recognitions. To straight power and the eagerness to use it.

Still—because he's new?—I ask him about something I saw recently.

"Do you see a ghost now?" He grins, smoker's teeth. Looks from side to side, puts big knuckly hands up beside his ears, wiggles his fingers. "Hello? Am I Casper?"

The conference rooms are unbelievably tiny. No more than closets really. Two chairs, a quarter inch between the knees, and the walls right there. Smaller than the smallest elevator. Like a womb you share with another fetus for an hour. Who had thought of it? On occasion, with the right person, the intimacy can be thrilling. To Rose, whose perfume fills the space, I said it was like two soul-moths, the wings grazing. She blushed and said you could say that. More often it is tense, fraught. Both of you talk rapidly to fill the space. And then, not infrequently, there is this. Two animals sewn into a pirate's sack. I zoom in on the ridges in his cords, the woebegone furrows between them.

"Give me more of that," he growls, chin angled up.

More of what? We'd been sitting in silence, the soup curdling in. "Hello?" I hear, and throw myself further into it, wading into the tough talk like a surf that will wake or pulverize me. "What about—?" And I ask him about some events over the years, the ones I'd come to call *transmissions*. Though I don't use that word with him.

"Ideas of reference," he says.

"Ideas of reverence,"[9] I murmur. Clearly enough that I hear the difference, but not loudly enough for him to catch it. *Echolalia* and *Perseveration* are words that appear often in my chart. Pat, a fat nurse who likes to start things, showed me one night.

Now he's standing, his ass in my face. A juicy fart would be the perfect ending. He turns the doorknob, lets it roll back. Turns. His crotch at my eye, baggy brown pleats. I do a zoom and walk awhile in the furrows, turned earth, up and down. I look up. Moustache ends hanging out of red, hair, ceiling. Sometimes the goop clears when I least want it to.

_____

9 A certain class of synchronized movements, more intense than coincidence, has for me the character of dancing with a stronger and infinitely more accomplished partner. If you accept this stranger's outstretched hand, and try to follow steps that are fleeter and more subtle than any you know, you may find yourself swept into a ballroom of unimagined opulence, where you catch glimpses of jewels and finery, fantastic faces, that you can hardly believe exist outside of dream. Following such a lead means finding the utmost pliability and quickness of response within yourself: it is the willingness to be led, the eager abandonment to command, that lends to feet so ardent to mimic grace, grace itself. The dance lasts a second—an eternity. It is only when you find yourself again, breathless, in the seat you once occupied that you perceive the last wonder of the dance: it took up no span of your life and yet occurred within it; it spun you nowhere yet you are not where you were. A number of such paradoxes are folded tight inside one marvel, which you will carry like a locket at the centre of yourself, the astonishment and rippling curiosity of having danced with Time. Often the first chord of the music, the unknown hand stretched toward your table, resembles mere coincidence. Indeed, if it is regarded as such for more than an instant, the perfumed hand vanishes. Ardency is the first requirement in a partner.

He gives me a hateful look, a glare that promises he will make me a special project. And I think he must have followed through, because suddenly, very suddenly, like a rip of cold air, he is nowhere near me, ever. I see him standing down the hall, though not with his hands on his hips, not glowering. Not even looking up. As if he'd been yanked off me by someone very stern. Like one kid just windmilling into another on the ground, a teacher hauling him back by the shoulders. Rare, for all the bullying; the two people had to match exactly, like dancers. I don't know what all might have happened between us.

· · ·

I answered a knock on the door. Summer, early fall, 2007— afterward I told myself to write down the date, but I forgot to. My hair was greasy, I hadn't shaved or washed lately. It had been maybe a week since I'd left the apartment. "Good evening," said an elderly, egg-faced man. He didn't stare; no doubt he met all kinds, knocking on doors. A middle-aged woman stood beside and slightly behind him; she smiled politely. The man said he was from Elections Ontario. He had bright eyes magnified by thick lenses and was bald save for a monk's fringe of short white hair. During my enumeration, he paused when I gave my birth-date: August 15, 1955. He looked up from his clipboard with those large bright eyes and extended his hand. "August 15, 1937," he said. The Guernica year—seventy years before. We shook hands warmly.

I watched him walk down the hall with his younger lady companion. Feeling buoyed by the brief encounter, floating in it as in warm salt water where I need barely move my limbs. I watched them almost to the elevator. They did not knock on any other doors.

I understood him to be an emissary, an angel calling me gently back to myself.

. . .

On October 29, a song came into my head insistently. I hadn't thought of it in years, but now I heard it constantly. It was a song from my early childhood. I heard my mother's voice, clear and warm, but I couldn't see her face, she must've been behind where I lay.

> *I had a little nut tree,*
> *Nothing would it bear*
> *But a silver nutmeg,*
> *And a golden pear;*
> *The King of Spain's daughter*
> *Came to visit me,*
> *And all for the sake*
> *Of my little nut tree.*

I wrote down the words—the voice stopped singing then—and pinned them to the black foam board that covers a third of one wall of this room, from near the floor to above my head. The area involved is about thirty square feet. The notes on the transmissions since April covered the black completely, layers deep in places. I had to push the pin hard to make the new note stick. Looking at the mass of cards and pages and Post-its and magazine photos and newspaper clippings, I felt a mixture of security and mild dread. Like someone who has filled his pantry and fridge with groceries but knows that at some point it will all have to be cooked. It will be big, I thought. Long. It wasn't so much the number of transmissions as it was the gaps between them. I had the sense of something strong enough to stay half-hidden, to take its time emerging.

I typed "I had a little nut tree" into Google and saw a black-and-white picture of Catherine of Aragon, one of those northern Renaissance portraits I find so frustrating and moving. Their blend of awkwardness and sophistication, as if talent is coming into focus randomly, is what you find in paintings by gifted high school students, which convey an external likeness guilelessly, without any trace of a peculiar inner life. "The characters in the nursery rhyme," I read, "are believed to refer to the visit of the Royal House of Spain to King Henry VII's English court in 1506. 'The King of Spain's daughter' could be either Princess Juana or her sister Catherine of Aragon, daughters of King Ferdinand and Queen Isabella. The princess in the nursery rhyme was probably Catherine, who was betrothed to Prince Arthur, heir to the English throne. Arthur died and Catherine married his younger brother, King Henry VIII. The first of Henry's six wives, she was discarded by the King to make way for Anne Boleyn, whom the common English people called The Great Whore."

The song had a second verse I hadn't known. My mom never sang it.

> *Her dress was made of crimson,*
> *Jet black was her hair,*
> *She asked me for my nut tree*
> *And my golden pear.*
> *I said, "So fair a princess*
> *Never did I see,*
> *I'll give you all the fruit*
> *From my little nut tree."*

. . .

On November 2, I parked my car on the west side of the grounds of the former Hamilton Psychiatric Hospital. The buildings are being converted to office space for other social services. The work is proceeding from east to west, and the old brick buildings I parked beside, some of the original asylum buildings, are mostly deserted. I seldom run into anyone apart from an occasional dog walker as I roam the wide, grassy grounds. I strolled with my digital camera, looking for the right kind of tree, in sunlight, with dirt around its base. It was mid-afternoon and I kept glancing up at the waning sun. The light was hardly ideal for taking pictures, but I felt myself slowing down, and before the solstice shutdown, which I knew would come early this year, I wanted to shoot some versions of the marks Paul Tamburlaine had made, which had been in my mind since April. I found a stick to make my marks, and I found two trees in different areas. A pine tree, with low, bushy branches, in moist soil thick with fallen needles. And a maple tree, with no lower branches, in a circle of pale, cracked dirt. Neither was ideal, but each had features I liked.

The shutdown started soon after, and went remarkably fast. Inside a few days I could only read magazines, short articles with pictures, and soon after that, nothing at all. I couldn't follow the words with my eyes let alone understand them. If I got to the end of a sentence and tried it again, it was as if I was encountering it for the first time. Wisps of meaning clung around some words, but then dissolved into jots and squiggles. I stopped trying to read. Took as much time off work as I could. It is so much like that scene in 2001 when HAL's circuits are pulled out module by module. One function less as Dave Bowman moves along the row. The process might be even more radical now, the ruptures in functioning more extreme. All that's really changed in thirty-five years is my reaction to it. I fight it less. It's a small, huge change. Still, I panic and flail sometimes, lashing out like a disturbed sleeper, especially if I'm asked, or ask myself, to think decisively. (And in those instants of flailing I see how easily, without this modicum of understanding, the panic could transmute to pathology, to diagnosis and treatment, to catatonia or worse.) The best I can manage is to let go and allow myself to sink into this grey, weighted dream, like one of those divers being lowered into the dark, their senses sheathed, looking so cumbersomely languid as they take their slow-motion walks, tottering in dark fluid, giant babies on the ocean floor.

It lasts about six weeks. Thoughts of suicide come and go. I try to watch them calmly —these particularly dark, jagged-edged clouds—and remember that they have passed before. The amnesia is still almost total. But that *almost* is a giant gain. Dimly I remember that I have been here before. Entered and left. I remember that there was another side, without remembering what it was. I keep the space I wait inside small, tiny as I can. Drinking (too much, which is the enough I need), watching movies I have seen before. *The Sopranos* are a godsend, eighty-six hours I can visit and leave at will. The car with music is also good, this womb-corpuscle filled with the Clash, "Spanish Bombs" on repeat, down Duplex to Chaplin Crescent, travelling slowly up the bloodstream of Avenue Road, very late or very early (they are the same), when no one else, or only the occasional other, is awake.

. . .

One reliable source of comedy is to tell people exactly what you remember. True, it can cause suspicion in those not accustomed to considering single frames slashed from a narrative. It's not something they permit in themselves (or which, by now, is perhaps even possible), and their eyes imply you are holding out on them: *You went to Paris and you remember a Coke? An orange table?* But for others— sometimes easy to spot, sometimes found by surprise—there is, after a bewildered look, a bark of laughter, which sounds like pure relief, when they find that the main feature has been cancelled, something has overexposed or underexposed all that lavishly mounted celluloid, the projector's defective lamp has burned it white or left it black, and so you chat in the empty theatre lobby, the scheduled entertainment replaced by a wall sconce casting a muted oval, or the serial number plate of the popcorn machine and a corner of last month's poster pinned by a staple.

Even so. I'm haunted by the suspicion that I'm only trying to make a virtue of necessity. Don't most people remember their lives? It's not a question of elapsed time. My memories of my first trip to Europe, in autumn 1975, were no more abundant or coherent—I don't remember more abundance or coherence—thirty years ago than they are today. If I stopped relating to people the fragments I recalled, it was because their reactions could no longer distract me from the question behind the fragments: Where *was* I during my trip to Europe? Was I by then sunk so far into dream that events vanished as soon as they hap- pened, except for a few vivid flashes that jolted me awake and laid down durable traces? Or was it waking life that had become character-less, lacking an executive agent that would preserve tracks firmly? Depression is known to interfere with attention in numerous ways, including this one: perceptions reach the way station of short-term memory but fail to be committed to long-term storage. Experience penetrates no further than the file clerk's desk at the end of the day: Everything In Everything Out. *Just these few I couldn't find homes for, boss.*

Except—isn't there another possibility in that image? An overlooked one?

Can't *find* a home; not, there *is* no home. Think of the difference. "Don't look for a story in symptoms," one caseworker said. But where else would you look? Piece it out. Over the years, you laugh along with everyone: *Four months in Europe and that's all there is?* But maybe that's all there *was*. If you keep remembering the same few things, isn't that the opposite of random? Isn't it possible that those snippets *are* what happened? Are at least stepping stones to story? Like the pebbles Hansel dropped when nobody was looking, the ones that lead through the dark forest home.

· The chess park. Germany. Green grass for the dark squares, the light ones sprayed white. The chessmen stand thigh-high, like milk cans with handles on top to move them. A platform at either end, steps up to it, the player lounging on a chair with armrests. Calling out moves. Men beside the board, smoking, drinking coffee or beer, lift the piece and walk it to its new square. Or carry it off the board. The taken pieces on either side huddle like interested dwarves. A game ends, a lifter takes the loser's place. I think of

Hackney and Moose. I am out in Paul Tamburlaine position, by a shade tree off one corner, watching.

· More giantism. Frogner Park, Oslo. November: solid-grey skies, cold. Wandering among the life work of Gustav Vigeland—*The Human Family,* says a plaque in English. Huge figures in grey stone, the same grey as the sky, depicting men, women, children, singly and in groups. Massive grey limbs and torsos, simplified faces. Grey. The Gorgons' wasteland... Here there is a gap, *eine Lücke,* a fugue state probably, since there is not even fog or the dead-spool sense of elapsed time. It is the next instant, but I am far away. No idea where or how I got here. Panting, chest heaving—from running? Shirt soaked with tears, which are streaming down my face, off my chin. Vast Technicolor faces blooming in the sky. Weeping harder at the relief of colour. Line of people against a brick wall, the faces blurred. Keep staring up. Recognition comes seeping back: Liz Taylor. Rock Hudson. James Dean. *Giant.* Film. Another gap, *eine vollständige Lücke.* On the floor in my friends' room. They found me somewhere, brought me back to their hotel. Two days lying on my side, settled by the dark rectangle of air under the box spring. Coming back, slowly.

· In a hut at the tip of Sognefjord, a room with bunk beds. Playing cards at a table with three other travellers, a man and two women. At dawn the mail boat will take us up the fjord to the sea. My friends have headed south, to Paris. I am to meet them there in a week. They were reluctant to leave me, after Oslo. I'm all right now, better, I need to get my confidence back, etc. Really it was the instinct to crawl away. I don't want witnesses for what will happen next. The other man, a balding Ottawan, quips to the plump brunette: "If I told you you had a nice body, would you hold it against me?" Her thin blond friend shoots me a look out of robin's egg eyes: Can you believe him? From the angle at which I receive her glance, fractionally broader than it should be, I realize that I have left my body and am positioned ahead and to the left of it. The difference is very slight; perhaps I have not left it completely. The smudge in my peripheral gaze, to my right and just behind me, is myself, my body. I check my position relative to the other players. Everything accords with the new coordinates. The brunette to my left slightly closer, the angle sharper. The man, directly opposite me before, now slightly oblique and slightly closer. I watch my hands play cards; they play as usual, though they look different, viewed from an angle never seen except in photographs. Later, in bed, the civil servant and the brunette snoring in tandem, a soft voice from the bunk above asks me to come up and massage her back. No, I tell her. Come up and rub my back, she says. No, I repeat. On the boat the next morning, the three stay in the cabin with the mail sacks. It is bitter cold. I stay outside, pacing the frost-slick deck. Through the window, the blonde shoots me a stricken, wet-eyed look. On the next pass, I see her hunched over, shoulders shaking. Her friend hugging her, consoling. The civil servant gives me a wink. I see my hands unzip a plaid sleeping bag, exposing a long white body, very thin, the hip bones prominent. Is it possible? I have no answer. I am back in my body now. Frightened, I visit the captain in the wheelhouse. I make chattering small talk. He shrugs in his heavy wool sweater, murmurs, "As high above, so deep below." Gesturing up at the rearing cliffs and down at the icy blue water. The fjord, so narrow, must be immensely deep; though it is 10 a.m. and we are half-way there, the sun has not even cleared the precipices yet.

· · ·

When my watch breaks down for good, in early May, a whole year after it first began to fail, I find a repairman in the neighbourhood. I wait a few days, I don't know why. It is not a matter, after all, of waiting to see if it will start again—a process that could be drawn out indefinitely—but of knowing that it is broken. How could I have forgotten that?

Y Phung Watch Repair, on Yonge Street, is one of those cubicles of space behind the small windows you glance up at from the street and wonder what goes on, who lives, behind them. I climb a wide stone staircase with oak handrails, the stairs bowed from the weight of climbing bodies, thousands of them, over decades.

The repair shop is a tiny model of economy. Like a cell in a hive. The repairman works at a cluttered desk, just enough floor for his swivel stool to move back two widths of itself, wooden shelves and compartments on all four sides stuffed with parts and order slips. A dusty window looks out on the smart shops below, the corner of a blue crane constructing a condo in the distance. How long, tinkering with time, has he seen them come and go?

I hand my watch through the window. The hands have not moved from 2:22. He sits on his stool and I sit on a plastic chair on my side, my knees grazing the partition. After a time I stand up and watch him at work. Through the window over his shoulder, dust-blurred views of spring shoppers, faces hurrying in the sunny street.

A feeling of peace suffuses me. As if I am sunk in a warm bath sipping an espresso, the body limp and soothed, the mind alert. I wish I could prolong the moment and imagine paying to watch him work, ostensibly as research for a profile I will write. Recently I did such a profile of a painter friend, a write-up of the month I spent watching him work on a portrait, but in this case it seems too weird. Shyness stops me. (Though this desire, to get close to people as they work, grows ever stronger. I often find myself standing near the silver-haired produce manager at Longo's as he discusses fruits and vegetables with customers, feeling calmed and utterly absorbed.)

He recommends replacing the works with a cheaper Japanese model that will work at least as well. I agree and ask unnecessary questions to prolong the encounter.

He writes his guarantee in black pen on the back of his business card. *May 17 2008. Citadel. Miyata 2035 replaced. 1 year warranty.*

He wears three watches on his left arm, and glances at one or all of them to set mine. He hands it to me. The hands still say 2:22, but the second hand is running again. *No time elapsed.* I stare at it until it ticks over to the next minute.

Down on the street, I stand on the pavement in the sunlight. People pass in either direction, walking briskly, intent. Spring again.

Let's go home.

It is the last transmission, I think. Or know rather, as with the stopped watch. This dance with time has ended.[10]

. . .

I came back from Europe in December 1975, sure that it would be over soon. The ruptures were becoming too frequent, and too long-lasting. Disjunctions that had been intermittent for years were settling in, like a graft that finally overtakes the shoot, or a tumour that envelops an organ. Metaphor roved constantly to suggest something that eluded words. Slippages, I called them. Windows; then doors. One day I would reach The Door. The Door would shut behind, or I would wander too far away and not be able to find it again.

---

10 If I ever glimpse the true subject of a piece of writing, it is only a fleeting recognition; in fact, that fleeting glance tells me that I have reached the end of that project. The moment is like the gesture of a mysterious and recurrent partner at the end of a masked ball, who, just as he is stepping into the night, face half-turned away, lifts his mask for an instant, as if to say, mischievously, This is who you kept sensing nearby, in all that swirl of sound and figures...Who else?—or else to offer some hope of a faster recognition when we meet again.

It had to be soon. My job, as I saw it, was not to hasten it, since it was coming to meet me on its own schedule, but to avoid unnecessary delays. That thought obsessed me: how to let unfold, how not to impede. This waiting was the most painful and fantastic feature of the process. How was it possible that, for years now, I had been slipping in and out of phase, finding myself in one world then another, or increasingly in a grey, milky inter-zone, while still retaining as much ability to function as I had? I knew that functioning was the enemy, it was the only thing I was sure of. Breakdown, absolute cessation, was needed. But it couldn't be rushed. It was the culmin-ation of necessary stages; so how—besides this horrible waiting—to arrive at it?

Of what was coming, *it*, I had not much notion. Like another universe, it couldn't be imagined from where I was. I knew it would require my death—a death of some kind. The biography I had known, myself as a person, was approaching a termination. That was all I knew for cer-tain. What, if anything, might begin on the other side of that line was as unknown as the life of an egg and sperm cell approaching each other.[11]

---

11 At times I thought the death approaching would land me in art, the life of an artist I felt destined for but barred from by lack of ability. I had a facility with words, an ability to spin fantasies that made people laugh or wince, but I did not connect verbal production at the poles I practised it—wild talk, tame school essays—with literature. The novels I read were controlled hallucinations, not staccato bursts of whimsy or dutifully stitched reports. I had read a bit on lucid dreaming, and I thought that art in that sense might end my confusions. I would not wake up, but like the lucid dreamer I would develop the ability to enter my own dream with the

I worked a year at Stelco, in the coke ovens. Dodging so many perils in the steel company underlined what I already knew: accidental death was not what was approaching. The charge car, the prow of a black ship, loomed out of smoke and I dove, so close it clipped my airborne boots. That happened many times. A man was crushed to hot jam between an oven and its huge door. People gave me pills, coloured capsules, and I took them, standing between the billows of purple-green gas and the roaring columns of flame. Inevitability grants immunity. When the destination is unalterable, "digression" loses all meaning.

I smelled a strange, elusive smell, a bit like burning hair. I realized I had smelled it faintly for months, maybe years, but it was stronger now. Showering and showering didn't remove it. It hid in my nostrils behind the soap. The scent would disappear, then return. A brain tumour? I had heard of such a symptom, I thought. But no, it would not be that.

I switched universities, going to York in Toronto. Maybe it was there. Maybe I had to move around, meet it somewhere. I rented a damp and mouldy basement apartment in Willowdale. The Geists, my upstairs landlords, argued

semi-control that is sometimes reported as a voice saying: "This is a dream. You can direct this." I did not see a prospect of waking once and for all, nor of ending the confusion between waking and dreaming, but art might offer a middle way: a way of infiltrating dreaming-waking with enough form that it acquires a richness of meaning irrespective of its ultimate reality. Though I came to discount lucid dreaming, and even despised myself for believing in it, I now see that it offered a viable analogy. A rough blueprint that I have spent the last thirty years stumblingly refining.

incessantly night and day, an opposition so unrelenting it seemed incredible that a couple still in their thirties had achieved it. Hiss to squabble to tirade: all-hate, all-the-time. I made a plywood table and spray-painted it lime green, my lungs stabbing for days afterward from the fumes in the unventilated space. Dinner was always tuna stirred into Campbell's cream of mushroom soup, heated and served over Uncle Ben's rice.

As at McMaster, I attended classes fitfully. I would take my seat in the back, the professor looking up in surprise, then spend the class trying to remember how I'd got there. A bus ride? Walking? Nothing. Words ran together, blurring into a grey paste that put me to sleep, but sometimes they popped clear in luminous relief. The Autopilot wrote essays and exams. My seminar leader, a graduate student who resembled a young Ayn Rand, detested me, her grimaces and sarcastic comments making this so clear the other students looked away in embarrassment. She gave me C- and C+ on my two big papers. Put-downs in red ink filled the margins. But those essays had been done, not by The Autopilot, but by myself in a luminous phase, excited and buzzing with ideas. That is what impelled me to do what I had never done in seventeen years of schooling: complain to the instructor. The professor looked at the papers, frowning. "I'm sorry," she said. "It's not right. But we switch sections after Christmas"—she raised her eyebrows—"if you can hang on till then." She gave me A+ on both essays I wrote for her. After the first, she

took me aside to say it had nothing to do with restitu-
tion, making up for, she wouldn't do that; and, after a
half-page appreciation at the bottom of the second, on
Marvell's "The Garden," she broke off to say, "Really, I
am filled with admiration."

Annihilating all that's made
To a green thought in a green shade.

At this success, an alternative flickered—nothing so
concrete as a goal or even a wish, but a glimpse, a peripheral sheen, of a path that led successfully out into the
world of a career and other people. A vista, a prospect,
opened up, another way, just for a second, until I remembered the other thing waiting for me. Like conversing with
an attractive woman, an interlude in a coffee shop, before
remembering you're late for dinner with Mrs Geist.

In German class the professor told me I had been
nominated for a Goethe Institute scholarship. I could
study in the Black Forest for the summer, if I wanted.
Considering it for a day or two, I tried to squint inwardly
to see The Autopilot, whom I knew only by his actions.
Usually I resented him as the master of useless delays who
was dragging the process out, inflicting greater pain. But
now I had to wonder: Could he be part of it too? He had
done the work that won the scholarship, obviously. Could
that mean—

Yes, I decided. Maybe...

It will happen in Germany, I thought. Feeling more and more certain.

The blue pool. Blaubeuren, where I stayed in the summer of 1977, is a small town in the Black Forest region of southern Germany, *in der Nähe von Ulm* in the soft local dialect. Its chief attraction, the source of its tourist economy, is the Blautopf (the Blue Pot), a large round pool of deep-blue water fed by a spring that is a relic of the last ice age, when the Danube flowed from Ehingen over Blaubeuren to Ulm. The water is so clear you can see down twenty metres to the bottom, down to where the sides begin to slope like a funnel; it seems you are seeing deep into the earth. A cornucopia of deepest blue. It is the last day of January as I write this, the coldest day of the year so far, and the sky is a pale porcelain echo, thinned and faded over thirty years, of the limpid sapphire I remember. Yet the colour behind my eyes is the same. And I can still hear the gasps and groans wrenched from people seeing it for the first time. Each new visitor would circle the viewing walkway, a rather brutal construction of slatted grey steel, before settling on a spot, always at the maximum distance from anyone else present, to lean on the metal railing and stare into the blue depths.

I checked into a gasthaus recommended by the Goethe Institute, where several other international students were staying. Frau Kächele, the proprietor, was a crisply pleasant widow whose constant soft humming seemed to emphasize the silent efficiency of her house, like the overhead buzz of a power line in a still summer field. The Autopilot was also working efficiently, and my two months of German studies constituted the most sustained attention I had given to schoolwork in several years. Finally, I felt I understood The Autopilot's role, and my resentment of him vanished. I had overestimated his powers and underestimated his importance. He had a job to do, vital but limited, and almost completed now; he receded in my mind as a cog, about to become an anachronism. His function had always been implicit in his name: he would be switched off when he needed to be. I had blamed him for delays, but he had no such powers. Perhaps, like a good clerk, he even facilitated matters above his station, clearing the decks so that the key players could operate. These now stepped forward and announced their names. I was allowed to know some of their functions. More would become clear to me later, during the fall. I had the impression of a (perhaps ironic) play before the play, in which the actors introduce themselves and give précis of their roles, then bow and disappear to wait for their cues.

More dependable lighting helped my studies. Now that the fluctuations in my visual field had eased, I realized how badly they'd hampered my concentration. The light was even now, though a bit too bright. When I awoke at 6 a.m., after a few hours' sleep, the light in the room matched the light beyond the window: full and shining, like noon. After classes ended in the afternoon, I took a very long walk, in a different direction each day, trying to tire myself out enough to sleep that night. Whether walking or studying, I felt so tireless that I took breaks at intervals I assigned myself rather than from actual fatigue. This bubbling energy, constant like the Blautopf, was strange but highly pleasurable, even thrilling. I tested it sometimes. Dropping to the floor beside my bed to do fifty push-ups, then, after a minute getting my breath back, repeating the set. I had to do many sets before my arms began to wobble. Hitting that wall was hard work, and a bit unnerving, so I stopped trying.

The social life with other students was easy, and problematic. Visiting with them in cafés or their rooms, I was talkative, even ebullient, cracking jokes in the fractured mix of French, German and English that we used. I was aware of contributing more than my share to the camaraderie. That, too, made a welcome change from recent years. There were slippages, though, as if The Autopilot—if it was The Autopilot—wasn't as reliably programmed for social encounters. At the morning break, Edwin from the Philippines or Carlos from Peru would approach me, grinning, eager to share a laugh about the night before. And I wouldn't remember anything about the joke they told again, even though I was often credited with having made it. When I laughed along with them, sometimes catching shards of recollection that could have been half-confabulated, spliced from other meetings, they looked uneasy, perhaps because my face was briefly a complete blank before these routines kicked in. It wasn't drink; we sipped tea more often than beer, and besides, alcohol had as little effect on me as push-ups. After a few weeks they invited me along less often, and when they did, I begged off on the excuse of studying. Top marks, I said, were a prerequisite for continuing my program back in Canada. They nodded sympathetically; most of them were vacation students, children of businessmen whose firms had clients or suppliers in Germany.

A fixed part of my routine was multiple daily visits to the Blautopf. Usually I was alone—the students didn't return after their first day—and this was always true on my first visit in the morning, killing time before Frau Kächele opened her breakfast room at seven. The ends of the metal walkway didn't quite meet; they formed an incomplete circle, like a horseshoe. At one end, under a peaked roof, was a painted diagram of the spring and pool, what we could see above ground and the aquifer and channels we couldn't see, below. On a shelf below this were brochures with photos of the blue pool and the town, and a write-up in three languages of the Blautopf and its *Urquelle,* or secret source. Across from this, at the other end of the walkway, was a shed with a padlocked door. I assumed it contained the controls for the sluice gate on that side, over which the pool brimmed and splashed to form a stream.

One morning the door to this shed was open, and a little man with a huge head was standing with his back to me, turning a wheel. The proportions of his head and body, and the disproportion between them, were extreme. His head was half again the size of a normal adult head, but his body was the size of a five-year-old's. He did not look like any dwarf I'd ever seen. A stiffness in his posture suggested age, or injury, but the tiny wrists and hands poking out of his sleeves—the only parts of his body I could make out in his baggy clothes —looked smooth and babyish; yet they were turning the wheel, which was fully half his size. He didn't give any sign he knew I was there, but I was sure that he did. I felt a prickling in my stomach, a spiny tickling. Still, despite my unease, I went about checking for perceptual distortions, as I had been doing for years. I moved to various places on the walkway, but his proportions didn't change. They weren't due to any trick of light or perspective I could discover. It was strange how he never paused in his work. His unhurried constancy was one of the queerest aspects of a sight I was finding more and more oppressive.

From a point midway around the walk, I stared down into the blue pool. Its colour changed in three distinct stages, without gradations between them, like the layers in a Jell-O dessert: a swimming pool green near the surface, then a darker aquamarine a couple of metres down, then the deep sapphire of the bottom half of the bowl. When the guidebooks talked about the piercing blue, they were really talking about the layer at the bottom. I looked up and saw the tiny man standing beside a tree, looking at me. He was well back from the pool, I couldn't make out his features. Just the large pale oval of his face next to the tree. He had one of his hands on the tree's trunk; a pale smudge, like a moth that had landed on the bark. Neither of us moved. I thought of a gnome in a Grimms' tale. Then I thought, with a gush of nostalgia that brought me to the point of tears, of Paul Tamburlaine. I felt a sudden intense longing not just for Paul but for a time before him, for my earliest childhood, for the years I had a few scattered memories of and for the time before that, the first long, blank wave, unknowable to me, that had spent itself at Paul Tamburlaine, he stood like a marker at the end of it.

I turned and walked quickly away. Though I stayed away from the Blautopf a few days, and approached it cautiously the next time, I wasn't really afraid of seeing The Regulator again. I had a strong sense of the rhythm of occurrences, whether they were likely to be singular or repeating. And though certain events were predominantly visual, they struck me as a kind of protolanguage, utterances that were both sufficient in themselves and part of a larger pattern. In this case, he had said his piece.

The course ended in late July and the students dispersed to their home countries. I stayed on in Frau Kächele's house, sometimes the only guest, but more often with her usual trade of two or three tourists. My walks lengthened prodigiously: fifteen, twenty, thirty kilometres and more. Partly it was to fill the time that school had filled, and partly to try to find the elusive tiredness that would make me sleep. Sleep had shrunk to about two hours a night. One night I miscalculated and walked out too far to make it back before Frau Kächele locked the door at midnight, so I kept walking and entered her breakfast room at 7 a.m., as if just coming downstairs from a refreshing slumber. After that, I stayed out every three nights or so, enjoying the different look of places in the dark, though I avoided the blue pool, from an instinct that The Regulator would not permit a nighttime visit.

Frau Kächele seemed as crisply pleasant as ever, but one afternoon she knocked on my door and asked how long I would be staying. I was lying on my bed with my hands folded on my chest, a half-hour daily quiet time I had imposed on myself since I was sleeping so little. I said I wasn't sure but not past the end of August, since I had to return for school. *"Ist mir egal,"* she said, smiling, but her eyes looked cold. *Mir egal* was an expression that puzzled me. Literally, it's "equal to me" (either way), it doesn't matter; but when local people said it, usually in a chirping voice with averted eyes, it sounded more like: I don't give a shit. Or: Fuck you. She closed the door and walked away, humming. Her humming sounded louder now, perhaps because the house was so quiet.

I planned my trip to Dachau to last three days and to involve as much walking as possible. There would be two huge tramps at either end, with a train ride in between from Ulm to Munich. I had a list of cheap hotels and *Fremdenzimmer,* but I thought it more likely that I would make do with naps on the train and by the side of the road, which turned out to be the case.

Dachau itself did not make a deep impression on me. The former concentration camp had an air of terrible sadness, but almost worse, it seemed completely evacuated, abandoned despite its visitors, as if history had utterly spent a place, used it up like Kleenex and moved on. I reached it on foot after walking out from Munich and, without intending anything dramatic, I found myself walking along the former train line, its ties and rails half-buried by wan, sickly grass. Ahead of me, I saw buses parked and people staring in my direction. I felt self-conscious, and mystified that I was attracting their interest. As I walked around the display, I noticed a woman, pale, with short grey-blond hair that curled in front of her ears like commas. I had seen her before; she was a guest at Frau Kächele's. Now she appeared on first one side of me then the other, then right in front of me, her position changing with a suddenness that seemed impossible unless I was gapping out again, going somewhere between her appearances. What's more, I always saw her face in profile and in a strangely flattened perspective, as if she were the Queen on a playing card. I moved around in my checking way, but her face kept its angle and flatness with respect to me, yet without any apparent movement to counter mine. The faces of the other tourists looked normal, though they blurred if I stared at them. It was like a scene constructed with only one reliable element, the rest ad hoc and liable to dissolve. The lighting was dim, too, I noticed now. Far dimmer, that grainy dusk, than even discreet museum lighting should allow.

I went outside to escape it. I walked off the tarmac of the parking lot and sat down by the train tracks I had walked in on. It was a hot August day, the insects buzzing. I opened my notebook and began describing a coffee shop I had been in yesterday. These notebooks had been part of both trips to Europe, a traveller's accessory which I wrote in sporadically. I had no interest in keeping a diary, and though for years now, since giving up the piano, I had regretted the lack of an art form in my life, I knew that writing could be no substitute for music or, especially, painting. The sentences I took down were like captions, notes in lieu of the scenes I wished I could paint in luscious oils. Sometimes this note-taking had a side benefit, though. Once described, a Vision, as I called the most vividly recurring scenes, would become more muted; its colours softened and I saw it less often. This damping tactic, which I was half ashamed of, seemed regrettable but convenient. Another benefit of the notebook was that it gave days that were very gappy a more solid feel; I could flip back through pages of blue ink and feel the described scenes connect to each other in a way that made *me* feel more solid, minimizing the spaces between the entries, which amounted really to most of the time, and privileging these recorded instants. I had always known books to have this property, of course; I had used it very consciously in the last few years. A very tattered week, a mixture of fog and gleams, could be held together by the simple block of *Crime and Punishment*: the holding of it in your hand, an appreciable chunk, and making your way through it, chapter by chapter. It was just a surprise to find that my own words could serve the same purpose, and do so, I was beginning to suspect, even more efficiently.

The Grey Lady was walking through the field, well away from me and from the tracks. She was wearing a white blouse, untucked. When a breeze filled it briefly, it gave the effect of a nightdress. I heard words and cocked my head to the right to hear them better.

a doll drifts through the high grass
seeking a little girl

I didn't like the words when I read them back. They didn't satisfy as description and they didn't satisfy as poetry. On the other hand, they were what I had heard. I liked that, that connection. It made me feel more of a piece. As if there was more to me. I wondered if such a connection could be honed, sought out. But then the thought bored me, or it discouraged me so deeply that it became bore-dom. The dream of art had been a long and intense one, a hope I had retired with great difficulty. I didn't want to reawaken it.

On the way back, after walking for several hours, I stopped by the side of a road and looked out over a wheat field. With a shock that seized my heart in my chest, I realized I had reached The Door. I was standing right in front of it. It came as a complete shock, because I had been walking along dully for hours, listless in mind and spirit. Times over the years when I have tried to describe what followed, it has always come out wrong and has led to unpleasant, sometimes drastic consequences. Depending on the listener, my account has been understood as a mystical vision, a psychotic hallucination, or simply a terribly vivid dream that I mistook for waking reality. Each listener has responded differently, though in all cases vehemently, the description has been accurate to that degree. So having erred so often in trying to describe the indescribable, I will say only this this time. Two mistakes I'd made were corrected instantly as I gaped at what was before me. I had worried that I might not recognize The Door when I saw it. What if, with all my gaps and fogs, I missed it somehow? Now I realized there had never been any chance of that. The Door's singularity precluded it. It was like nothing I had ever seen or imagined—like nothing but what it was. Also, I had always assumed that, when I got there, it would be terrifying—but its reality was utter, radiant joy. This was not an expulsion, it was pure admittance. (Terror and expulsion, I would learn, were simply the other side of joy, the same radiance bent and scattered.)

Still, for all the pulsing jubilance whirling inside me, there was a moment when permission was asked and granted. I felt it clearly. It was like the moment in a marriage ceremony when the conducting official spells out the meaning of the coming union and the participants must perceive the articulated conditions and consent to them. In some quiet place within a storm of celebration, I was reminded that there could be no return from this point— and reminded that I had long known this, so there could be no question of being duped in a frenzy—and, to the extent that I was still capable of choosing, I chose freely, feeling myself enter.

(Was it a real choice? Even when I have cursed myself for making it, I have had my doubts. I imagine someone stuck in a dim puppet theatre who sees a panel in the wall slide open to reveal the bounty of a city street in sunlight. While he is gaping at the scene, a voice reminds him that he is free to forgo the dangers outside, the door can be slid shut and the jerkings of the marionettes in the dusk resume. In what real sense is that a choice?)

At some point I fell down and, it seems, lost consciousness for a time. Throughout the experience my eyes were under great strain, struggling to follow an onrush of rapidly changing colours and forms as well as shifts in scale and depth of field. A flattened, sky-wide frieze of huge geometrical forms, rectangles of electric blue and rhomboids of liquid gold and chocolate brown, would give way abruptly to a close-up of seething molecules, gold-tan corpuscles like the fat globules in a rich gravy, rushing and jostling under a sheer tubular skin. The only constant was the wide open aperture, as if my pupils were dilated to the maximum, flooding my eyes with light (while keeping all views sharp as an acid etch), until finally—it might have been a minute or an hour later—the electric blue began to tilt sideways, slowly at first and then more rapidly, whorls of dark fur narrowed the visual field in spiral bands, like the sphincter of a shutter closing, I felt myself tipping in the direction of the blue, and I felt, in a muffled, distant way, points of my body thump as I blacked out.

When I opened my eyes, I saw fuzzy white-grey shapes and thin green columns. They started next to my eye and went into the distance. Slowly, I realized they were pieces of gravel with grass blades growing between them. It was a relief to see such plain, familiar things. They rested me, and I lay on my side a long time looking at them.

I got up carefully. My shoulder and knee were throbbing where I'd hit, and my right ankle was tender, but nothing seemed broken. I made my way slowly along the side of the road, on a strip of pale dust between the road and the gutter. I felt subdued. A bit stunned, and very sober; aware that, at the moment, I needed some time that was as uneventful as possible to recover. I walked in the direction of Blaubeuren, keeping my head down, watching my feet shuffle forward, raising little puffs of dust that settled again.

I was a while realizing I wasn't alone, and probably hadn't been since Dachau. Raising my eyes from my feet, I saw that the rustlings and flittings I had taken for birds were in fact the rapid movements of The Grey Lady,

appearing on one side of the road then the other. She
wasn't walking or running through the high grasses but
rather hovering and flitting just above them, with erratic
flutterings reminiscent of a butterfly's. I took her in in
glances, guided by a new sense of economy not to study
her too closely. She had the waxy, flattened face, the playing card profile, about the size of, or just a little smaller
than, a normal head, with a body of about the same size
below it, grey-white and vaguely birdlike, with two stubby
appendages that did not look like wings or arms and in
any case didn't move in her dartings. *The Grey Lady.*
There seemed a danger in using names that made all the
Players sound like humans, even those that were clearly
not. I told myself I should guard against it.

I walked along with my head down, thinking about
that. The Grey Lady left for a time. Then she was back, a
startling blur right beside my face. Seeming to sense my
fright, she moved farther away—her manner of movement weirdly fluid, as if she were sliding on tracks in the
air—and, keeping pace with me, just visible in the corner
of my right eye, she started a conversation, or rather
resumed one it seemed we were already having.

Not as you are. It was a woman's voice, soft and low, but
with a buzzy undertone, faintly machine-like.

I can't wake up.

No.

I can't get back.

No.

I'm only awake when I'm bored. It sounded odd as I said it, yet it seemed true.

I recounted some instances in support of it, which she listened to without comment.

You can direct this to a degree.

How?

She didn't answer, and receded from my sight, so that I thought she had gone. Then she was back, sliding up almost parallel again.

By coming back? I asked.

Going back.

From here?

That's the past already.

We talked in this way a while longer, a cryptic-companionable exchange that relaxed me even as it confused me slightly, and then she dropped back and I knew somehow that she would not appear again on this walk.

I entered Frau Kächele's house furtively, trying to get past the breakfast room and up the stairs without being seen. On one of my recent walks I had lost my watch, but I knew that it must be after seven, though perhaps not long after. Frau Kächele would rather you missed breakfast by hours than mere minutes.

But Frau Kächele herself was sitting at a table, smoking. Smoking was not permitted in her house—signs were posted to that effect—and I had never seen her smoke. Yet she was taking the deep, relaxed drags of a habitual smoker, smoke drifting around her head, an ashtray heaped with butts on the table. She motioned, with her usual chilly courtesy, for me to take the seat across from her.

"You're not—" Suddenly I could not remember the German for "humming," though it was one of the first words I had looked up in her house.

"Humming and smoking, they're the same, *ja?*"

I laughed and said that, though I had never considered it before, that sounded exactly right. I was relaxing in this exchange, relieved to feel the tension I had always felt in my landlady's presence beginning to dissipate. It went beyond relief to a sense of complete well-being I felt suffusing me, a fellow feeling I had not known for a long time. A gaiety, bubbling in my chest, at the certainty that human beings, even dissimilar personalities, could always find common channels to flow and mingle in. Frau Kächele was smiling with tightly pressed lips, as if at a joke she could barely suppress.

"Liesl?" I said, in a voice hushed with wonder.

She smiled openly, but did not answer directly the intuition that had flown into my head. "I came to Germany a long time ago. You know that perfectly well," she said tartly.

It was true, I did seem to remember having heard that. It was one of the million things I had known and then forgotten.[12]

---

12 A continual surprise in writing is the shaping power of the forgotten, partner of the remembered. Another (the last?) thing stolen by the Close Thief, forgotten until a late revision of this, was my paternal grandfather's gold pocket watch.

She now caught me up on the missing years, which, she regretted to say, had been consumed mostly with a battle against ill health. Her face, puffily middle-aged and more crafty than intelligent, did not resemble Liesl's at all, but in one of the amazing scenes in the dream, one I remembered very clearly, we had been sitting side by side on our couch, peering at our pictures in the high school yearbook and marvelling with rueful chuckles at how thoroughly the years had misconstrued our looks. She suffered from a rare medical condition, she explained to me, which complicated her life with a social ineptness she could only manage by means of stereotyped routines that limited and made predictable her interactions with people. To put it bluntly, she was missing her amygdala, or rather it was so atrophied as to be useless. The amygdala was the almond-shaped organ in the brain that enabled the recognition of fear and anger in other people's faces. Without a timely sensing of these negative emotions, a person could not help but step on toes constantly, speaking and behaving inappropriately and driving others away.

I interrupted to say I knew of this condition, I had read of it.

"I know you know of it," she said with her un-Liesl-like brusqueness. "That is precisely why we are talking now."

When she had finished her account, including many unsuccessful medical treatments, and her deliberate choice of a lifestyle that would allow for busy interaction without involvement, a kind of hiding in plain sight, I expressed sympathy for all that she had been through, and admiration that she had managed it alone.

"*Bestimmt nicht!*" she blurted, straightening with affront. "*Ohne meinen Mann...*"

Following the gaze she flicked to a side table, I had an inkling of what I would see a moment before I saw it. The tiny legs, like sticks in a child's pants, with miniature workboots at their ends, dangled between the chair edge and the floor. Thankfully, The Regulator's head was hidden behind the *Speisekarte* Liesl supplied for those who wanted something more than the continental breakfast that came with their room.

"All he does is eat," Liesl said fondly, with a drag that burned a third of her cigarette.

Along the counter near The Regulator stood the three wicker baskets of rolls and foil-wrapped cheeses and various jams, none of them looking as if they had been touched. Looking back at his table, I noticed a notebook and pen beside one little hand.

"I don't want to be a writer," I said, with rising revulsion.

Liesl shrugged, butting out her cigarette. "Who does?"

A little after that, I reached the trimly typical house, with its white stucco walls, green-trimmed windows hung with flower boxes, the small square of shorn grass enclosed by a low black wrought-iron fence. I opened the front door as quietly as I could. The house seemed empty.

The breakfast room cleaned up and set for tomorrow's breakfast.

As deserted as the house seemed, I mounted the stairs carefully, trying not to make the slightest creak. At the turning was a mirror and I took a full look from close up, something I hadn't dared in years. The front of my T-shirt was streaked with brown and green, ground-in horizontal smears, as if I had been rolling back and forth in the dirt. At my temple and along one cheek were crusts of dried blood and pitted places, from the gravel.

This is it, then.

The face in the mirror nodded grimly, then grinned. The expressions, especially the contrast between them, struck me as vile. I spoke sternly, as to a child beyond its depth.

It will be bad. Worse than you can imagine.

The face didn't respond.

In my room, I sat on the straight-backed wooden chair. The other pieces of furniture were a single bed and a nightstand. I should get home, I thought. It should happen there. My return ticket was still in the front pocket of my green army pack. There were a half-dozen objects, plus a change of clothes on the closet shelf, that needed to be put back in it. It would take me five minutes. It seemed as if there should be more to do. It didn't seem right somehow that I could snap my fingers and transplant the operation to another continent. That incongruity bothered me more than any other I had experienced lately.

I closed my eyes, my hands folded in my lap. It had been three days since I'd last slept, discounting catnaps on the train. Yet I felt a peaceful, bubbling energy flowing through me, around me and through me, as though I were immersed in a light electric current, humming like a tuning fork. I felt a fleeting fear of my own lack of fear. A momentary spike of awareness, far too slight to inspire action, that recognized utter lack of apprehension as a very bad state. A very dangerous one. The thought popped like a bubble, subsiding back into the morning's froth of well-being.

What seems the strangest, most unnatural thing, I thought, studying the perception like an unusually coloured pebble, is that I still don't feel tired, I can't get to where that is. Sleep is now a foreign country, and I can't get there from here.

ACKNOWLEDGEMENTS AND DEDICATION

The opening quotation from Augustine is taken from the 1993 edition of J.G. Pilkington's translation of *Confessions*, edited by Justin Lovill and published by The Folio Society, Ltd.

Thanks to Douglas Glover and his online journal *Numéro Cinq,* in which this work, in a slightly different form, first appeared.

Thanks to the whole talented team at Biblioasis for their commitment to book-making and for once again letting me fly my freak flag.

to the ones beyond the door

AUTHOR BIO

Mike Barnes is the author of twelve books of poetry, short fiction, novels, and memoir. He has won the Danuta Gleed Award and a National Magazine Award Silver Medal for his short fiction, and the Edna Staebler Award for his photo-and-text essay "Asylum Walk." His most recent book of nonfiction, *Be With: Letters to a Caregiver*, was a finalist for the City of Toronto Book Award and has been praised by Margaret Atwood as "Timely, lyrical, tough, accurate." He lives in Toronto.